SECRETS OF THE HAIR INDUSTRY

A Guide To Today's Booming Hair

Extensions Industry

First Edition

B DAKIN

Secrets of the Hair Industry
A Guide to Today's Booming Hair Industry

www.secretsofthehairindustry.com

ATTENTION SCHOOLS AND CORPORATIONS:
This book is available at quantity discounts with bulk purchase for educational, business, or sales promotional use. For information, send an email to
info@secretsofthehairindustry.com

Contents

Chapter 1: Hair, What to Wear

Just like a new outfit, a good pair of shoes, or a fresh lipstick color, the right hair or hair accessories can change your overall look and mood!

Human hair extensions have been around since the days of the ancient Egyptians, but not until the past 10 years have they really become a popular choice for the masses. Take a peek inside a local salon on any given day and you will see many people choosing hair extensions as a way of changing their hair style, adding length, or adding body and fullness to thin or thinning hair.

Women of all races are using hair extensions to add fullness and luxury to their heads and even women with adequate amounts of their own hair love to accessorize with hair extensions.

A popular choice for celebrities and everyday people, hair extensions can be used as a way to enhance our looks and our spirits!

Chapter 2: It's A Booming Industry!

Make no mistake about it, the hair extension industry is big business. The global demand for hair is growing and hair comes from many different countries and from people with varied backgrounds. The sources of hair may include women in India that are giving their hair to temples and women in Europe that are selling their hair for various reasons from needing the money for bills to being bored with long hair to raising money for charitable organizations.

In the United States there is an almost insatiable desire for hair of all types. Many high profile celebrities frequently wear hair extensions and several celebrities even have their own lines of hair extensions. While this luxury used to be a secret for the stars, the masses have been joining in at an incredible pace and the business is booming. Considering the celebrity culture, the decreasing cost of real human hair, and the new technologies that are available for applying the extensions this trend appears to have no end in sight.

It is interesting to note that while Americans spend an extraordinary amount of money on beauty and hair, many times the people giving their hair are not compensated. For example, thousands of Indian women give their hair in a religious act of piety at Indian temples. They visit the temples to give thanks or to deliver requests to the gods. Many of them have no money to offer the gods so the most valuable item that they possess is their hair. This process is called tonsuring and many of them have no idea that they are part of an exploding industry worldwide.

Chapter 3: What Do All Of The Terms Mean?

When discussing hair, hair types, hair applications, etc. there are many terms to consider. We have tried to break these terms down for you by providing short descriptions and answers below:

What is virgin hair?
Virgin hair is human hair that has never been chemically processed. By processed we mean colored, permed, etc.

What is Remy hair?
The term "Remy" can be a very confusing term in the hair industry. Remy hair can be virgin, processed (colored or permed), or unprocessed. Remy virgin hair refers to hair that is unaltered, with the cuticle still attached to the hair. Many would argue that Remy virgin hair is the best hair that you can buy. Hair which is of "non-remy" quality is sometimes referred to as "beauty supply store hair" and is relatively cheaper.

What is the hair cuticle and why is it important?
The hair cuticle is the outermost part of the hair shaft
and acts as a natural protection. This part of the hair is
responsible for the resilience and shine in hair. Virgin
hair that is 100% natural and free of chemicals has no
damage to the cuticles.

What is hair harvesting?
Hair is "harvested" to make extensions, wigs, and hair
pieces. Ideally, the hair strands are organized facing the
same direction from root to tip – hair might be cut close
to the scalp in a ponytail to achieve this. In other
harvesting techniques the hair is simply cut from the
head, gathered from the floor and packaged with no
regard for the way the hair strands are aligned. Since
hair whose cuticle layers are running in various
directions tends to become easily tangled, the hair is
then chemically processed. This process can damage
the cuticle layer and this type of hair is typically less
expensive. Sometimes this hair is even mixed with
animal or synthetic hair and may be referred to as "Yaki".

What is bulk hair?
Bulk hair is loose hair that is used for braiding, making
lace wigs by hand and other hair extension styles.

What does the term "weft" mean?
The type of hair used in weaving hair extensions is
called "wefted hair" and "wefting" is the process of
sewing hair together on the root side of the hair. Hair
strands are sewn across in a straight line, keeping it
freely hanging so that it looks like a hair curtain. Weft

hair is used for sew-in, glue and net weaving and when sewn in the weft is sewn onto the braided track of hair in the head.

What is the difference between a machine and hand-tied weft?

Hair wefts are made either by specialized sewing machines (machine weft) or by hand (hand tied weft). Machine wefts are made by sewing hair strands together with a specialized hair sewing machine. Hand tied wefts are made by hand tying hair strands around a strong weaving thread. For hand tied weft the cut ends are sealed by applying glue. Some think that hand tied wefts are thinner and lay flatter, making the hair look more natural.

What is the difference between single machine wefts and double machine wefts?

Single machine wefts tend to be thinner at the weft area and are made with a single layer of hair. Double machine wefts tend to be bulkier at the weft area, but because they are made with a double layer of hair they usually create a heaver, fuller looking weft.

What is weaving thread?

A thick thread especially made for weaving.

What are clip in, or clip on extensions?

These are extensions that are easy to attach, and this technique is the least permanent. Clip in/on extensions do not require the commitment associated with glued in extensions. These extensions are good for temporary styles that require more hair such as hair buns and pony tails, etc. Many times the hair weft has small hairpiece clips sewn onto them and when the wearer's real hair is sectioned, the clips are applied so that they are facing the scalp. These types of extensions are very versatile and should be removed before sleeping.

Chapter 4: How Are Extensions Applied?

There are many different techniques for bonding and sealing extensions. These techniques are discussed in greater detail below:

Bonding

Bonding is an approach to hair weave that lasts for a shorter period of time in comparison to a sew-in weave. This process involves the application of hair glue to a section of wefted hair then onto a person's natural hair and special hair adhesives are used in bonding to prevent damage to one's natural hair. This technique is quite common and it does not cause damage to the hair unless the wefted hair is taken out without proper directions from a professional. It is advised that weave bonding be installed for no more than 3 weeks because the glue begins to loosen up and lessens the attractiveness of the hair. There are 2 types of bonds: soft bond and hard bond. Soft bond is flexible and comfortable to wear and is made using latex, acrylic or silicone. Hard bond is the professional term for super glue. Hard bond adhesives last longer than soft bond adhesives because hard bond adhesives are not water based and therefore they do not fall apart. However, because the hard bond is rigid, the adhesives are not as comfortable as the soft bond adhesive. These bond attachments may generally last 4–6 weeks before a hair maintenance appointment is necessary.

Fusion

The fusion method delivers one of the most versatile and most natural-looking weaves. With this technique a machine similar to a hot glue gun is used to attach human hair extensions to individual strands of one's natural hair of about 1/8 to 1/4 inch squared sections for a fairly authentic look. Another option for fusion attachments is using hair which is pre-tipped with a keratin adhesive. A heat clamp is then used to melt the adhesive to attach the extension hair to the natural hair. Fusion weave allows for frequent washing hair and the use of regular hair products such as hair gels. However, this technique is very time consuming and it needs repositioning every 2-3 months as the natural hair grows. Also, because of the glue and the heat this method is more damaging to the natural hair then other methods.

Micro Rings (Micro Loops)

Micro rings or micro loops hair extensions use small metal rings (usually made of aluminium) lined with silicone with the extension hair attached. These are fixed to small sections of natural hair and tightened using a special tool that clamps the loop around the natural hair. The micro loops are designed to be small enough so that they are not visible in normal use. Micro loops need repositioning every 2-3 months as the natural hair grows and the micro loops move away from the scalp. Since this approach does not use heat or adhesives, these hair extensions usually cause less damage to the person's natural hair.

Netting

Netting is a technique which involves braiding natural hair under a thin, breathable net that serves as a flat surface onto which stylists can weave the hair extensions. This method requires the use of a hair net or cap to be placed over the person's hair that has been braided. Netting provides more flexibility than track placement because the stylist is not limited to sewing extensions to a braid. With netting there is the option of sewing the hair wefts onto the net or gluing. This technique is not as time-consuming as the other hair techniques.

Lace Fronts

Another development in weave extensions is lace fronts. Lace fronts are made from a nylon mesh material formed into a cap that is then hand-ventilated by knotting single strands of hair into the tiny openings of the cap, giving the hair a more natural and authentic continuity than typical extensions. The extension units can then be woven in or attached to a person's hairline with special adhesives. To ensure a proper fit, head measurements are taken into account with this type of weave. A lace frontal is best placed by a professional since more advanced weaving and hair extension techniques must be used. This method is popular because it allows the user to have access to a certain part of their scalp and at the same time it has an attractive, natural look.

Tracking

This is one of the most commonly used methods since it can be installed fairly quickly and it lasts considerably longer than the other techniques. However, this approach does not allow for regular hair maintenance. Tracking involves the braiding of a person's natural hair. In order to prevent the hair from being bumpy or uneven the hair is sewn horizontally across the head from one side to the other starting from the nape of the neck. The braided hair is sewn down and the hair weft extensions are sewn onto the braids. A weave can consist of a few tracks, or the whole head can be braided for a full head weave. With a full head weave, the braids are sewn down or covered with a net and extensions are then sewn to the braids. The number of tracks used depends on the desired look.

Chapter 5: Hair Types

There are many different types of natural hair extensions but the largest selection of hair extensions are made from either Indian or Asian hair.

Indian hair is the most popular hair globally and is the most highly regarded because of its durability, flexibility, and texture. Indian hair is naturally thick and lustrous, so it usually gives the best styling and installation options.

Asian hair is wiry and is typically somewhat coarse. Most Asian hair extensions are treated in acid bath that removes the cuticle. It is then further processed with silicone to give it an artificial shine.

Brazilian and Malaysian hair.....there is no such thing. Think about it.....in an image conscience area like Brazil would thousands of women shave their heads? If Brazilians did shave and sell their hair it would be very exclusive and very expensive – not marketed to the masses. Some companies choose to market hair as

"Brazilian hair" or "Malaysian hair" but it is really Asian hair that has been processed to appear to have more body. These terms may be used as a way for a supplier to market or classify a product but these are not pure terms that identify where the hair actually comes from. This hair tends to be less consistent in quality and texture than Indian and Asian hair.

Chapter 6: Your Hair Is An Investment -- You Get What You Pay For!

The demand for hair is high and today there are many places where consumers can buy hair. As discussed earlier in this book, there are different ways of harvesting hair. Be wary of non-virgin cuticle hair. Remember that this hair can be a collection of random hair that has been picked off the barber or temple floor and sometimes mixed with other hair that was left for trash after the wefting process was completed. The acid bath that this type of hair may go through destroys the hair cuticle and it is then dipped in silicone to cover up the imperfections. The hair will begin to tangle and mat after a few washes.

Virgin Indian hair is the most expensive hair that a person can buy but in the long run it is worth the initial investment. This hair is a better value and it will last longer. In its best form, this hair looks natural, can be cared for just like your own hair, and it can be used again in future hair installations.

Buying non-virgin cuticle hair ("beauty supply store hair") may save you money initially but in the long run you will spend more. Remember that with hair, you get what you pay for.

Chapter 7: Hair Care....Make It Last Forever (Or Almost Forever)!

Hair extensions offer versatility in styling and can be worn straight, curly, natural or dyed to the desired hair color. Good virgin hair is durable and will last six months up to a year. The longevity of the hair depends on how well the hair is maintained. Just as with a person's own natural hair, hair will be healthier and stronger when it is taken care of.

Treat your hair extensions like your own hair. Use good quality shampoo and conditioning products. To keep it in the best condition, you should wash and shampoo regularly using a quality moisturizing shampoo and conditioner. Hair extensions do not have the benefit of your own natural scalp oils, so adding natural oils (mink, jojoba, macadamia) will help to replace those necessary oils. To prevent dryness you may wish to apply oil twice weekly prior to shampooing and oils left on the hair overnight on the ends can be helpful. To straighten the hair, blow dry the hair and follow the drying process with a ceramic plated flat iron. Use oils and moisturizers to keep hair shiny, soft and manageable but stay away from products that contain alcohol since products containing alcohol will dry out the hair. You can also use products like gel and hair spray to keep the curls in place, but make sure to wash the hair frequently and do not leave gel and spray products in for a long time. Deposits from the hair products, if not washed off on a regular basis, can degrade the quality of the hair and combined with the use of heat can affect the smooth natural feeling and behavior of even the highest quality virgin hair.

Hair extensions may be colored and high quality virgin hair will handle the coloring process very well. However, remember that after you color or process virgin hair, it will no longer be virgin. We recommend consulting a hair professional for any hair coloring that is desired.

When combing the hair, always use an anti-static comb and start from the tips, working up little by little to the root. With the other hand, hold the base to keep it from shedding or causing tension at the roots.

When swimming in pools and hot tubs, it is best to wash hair right after swimming. If possible, avoid salt water since the salt can take the moisture out of the hair and the moisture loss will lead to tangling. Do not wear a swimming cap because the friction on the hair may cause the hair to mat. Because of the moisture stripping and tangling you may not wish to braid the hair when going into salt water. If you do braid the hair, braid the hair in only one braid at the back of the neck. Always remember to add a good leave in conditioner after swimming.

When sunbathing, braid the hair in one braid at the back of the neck and after sunbathing do not unbraid the hair until after the hair has cooled. Follow with the appropriate moisturizing shampoo and conditioner as needed.

When sleeping, make sure your hair is always completely dry when you go to bed. Sleeping on wet hair can mat and tangle your hair and over time may cause hair odor.

In general, when it comes to hair care, just remember that you have to care for your extensions just like your own natural hair. Brush your hair frequently and shampoo and condition your hair regularly, especially if you use a lot of hair products. If hair extensions are maintained properly, you will have smooth, tangle free hair for a long time and you will be able the reuse the hair many times.

Chapter 8: Hair Education

We hope that the previous chapters have educated you about hair extensions so you can make the proper choice for your hair needs.

Because of the growing demand for extensions there is also a growing demand for well trained extension stylists. Hair extension customers should do their research when selecting a quality professional stylist because a good stylist makes all of the difference. It does no good to have quality hair and then have it installed poorly or improperly. Make sure that you choose a stylist that has been professionally trained in the art of hair weaving and treatment.

Consumers and stylists alike can benefit from seeking as much education as possible in order to learn the hair types and methods that are most appropriate for a person's hair type and budget. Be careful about some of the information that may be available on the internet and make sure that you are receiving information from a respectable source. Many training materials are available in bookstores, through continuing education schools/companies, at hair/beauty conferences and in classrooms at cosmetology educational institutions. Also, it may be helpful to meet with successful professionals in the industry that can show you good hair techniques and share their own valuable wisdom and advice.

Chapter 9: If You Are In The Business, Do It Right

Are you currently running a business or thinking about starting a business in the hair extensions industry? The industry can be competitive but also very rewarding!

Perhaps you are considering becoming a supplier of hair extensions and "brokering" hair. The most important thing to remember is that having a solid consistent hair supplier is everything. Make sure that you are buying from a reputable supplier that can consistently provide good quality hair. If you are buying from overseas, many times you must pay upfront and wait several weeks for the hair to arrive. It is usually best to try to get a referral to an overseas supplier and be wary of some of the overseas suppliers that may offer to send you "samples". Unethical suppliers may send their best hair for "samples" and after you commit to a larger order and pay for it they send poorer quality hair. Even worse, sometimes the hair will arrive in its most unprepared form (dirty hair, hair containing lice, etc.). Hair buyer beware.

If you are brokering hair we really cannot emphasize enough the importance of taking your time to find a direct overseas supplier or a dependable U.S. based dealer that has a direct connection to an overseas supplier. This is sometimes the most difficult, time consuming, and expensive part of the process. Make sure that you are taking the time to find out the answers to some of the questions and topics we have discussed in this book. How is the hair harvested? If a local dealer is used then how many steps is that dealer away from the actual supplier/manufacturer? Does the dealer have influence over the supplier/manufacturer in the event that there is a problem with the hair order? All of this matters tremendously. If you do not do your research upfront and if you do not work with trusted hair sources then this will be an expensive lesson learned.

As a hair broker spend some time professionally marketing your product and always research the stores or stylists that you are selling hair to. While we recommend buying and using the highest quality hair possible, it might be necessary to sell Chinese hair if that is the only hair that will sell in your target market area. If you are doing "cold calling" to sell hair, remember to do your research before approaching a store or salon.....you would not want to blindly walk into a store or salon that focuses on natural hair care trying to sell hair extensions, would you? Save yourself the embarrassment by researching this in advance.

Are you a stylist or considering becoming a hair extension stylist? This can be a very profitable business because depending on the hair type, the time involved for installation, and the client needs, stylists can make hundreds, even thousands of dollars per hair installation.

If this is the case remember that your clients will continue coming to you for their hair needs and they will refer others that need your services if they find you to be trustworthy and reliable. Once you have created your "signature" in someone's head by installing hair properly, most clients will be associated with you for a very long time since they know that you are the best person available to uninstall the previous installation and this opens the door for you to create another hairstyle or install new hair. Education will be paramount since you will need to care for your client's hair just as your own. Making sure that you stay abreast of the latest trends and hair weave techniques will be a continuous process. Teach your clients to identify and purchase the best hair that they can afford and explain to them that quality is in the way the hair is harvested, not in how long the hair lasts. When your client's hair looks good this is the stylist's greatest reward. Always use the best hair care products and always recommend the best hair to your clients.

Maybe you are already an extensions stylist or a salon owner and you are looking to grow your business. Consideration may be given to adding to your existing stylist and salon services by actually providing the hair to your clients. Instead of allowing your clients to bring you "beauty supply store hair" for installation you can be the supplier of quality hair. This approach ensures that your best work can be done to please the client and selling hair can add additional revenue to your business.

If you are not sure how to start or where to start or how much money you need to start a business, do not over analyze this and get caught in an "analysis paralysis" loop. Just start! Jump in with whatever knowledge and money you currently have and go from there....this is a fast paced industry so time spent being fearful could be time better spent in business. This does NOT mean that you should move without educating yourself and without understanding the business and the related risks. In other words, you should not sit still doing nothing when even small steps in the right direction are better than doing nothing at all. For example, do not procrastinate in registering for another hair class if you are a stylist, do not wait to start researching quality hair suppliers and prices, do not hesitate in registering a new limited liability company if you are starting a business. You are already taking a positive step forward by taking the time to read a book like this one so that you will understand the hair extensions industry better. Congratulations to you!

Whether you are already in business or thinking of starting one the most important thing is to get organized. Here are a few tips to protect you and your company:

- Make sure that you keep your business and personal affairs separate by having a separate company structure and tax identification number (EIN)
- Open a bank account for the company and use it for all of the company's financial transactions
- Document in writing major transactions and business engagements
- Have all company business expenses billed in the name of the company
- Pay annual fees to the state and/or county in which you form the company and keep the company and business licenses in good standing
- Be careful about personally guaranteeing the debts or obligations of the company because your personal guarantee overrides the "business only"

liability. A personal guarantee cannot always be avoided (many credit card companies require a personal guarantee, for example) but be mindful of the implications

- Keep good accounting records and consider popular online accounting applications so that you can access your financial information from anywhere. Online applications also ensure that there are automatic and regular backups of your important data
- Find a good bookkeeper and/or tax accountant so that their expertise can be used in this area and you can focus on running and growing the business

Chapter 10: Summary

The goal of this overview was not to present everything there is to know about the hair extensions industry but to provide some general information to help the reader make the right choices in hair type and application technology to fit the individual's desired needs. Along the way it is our sincere desire that you enhanced your current knowledge and/or learned something new. Thank you for reading!

www.ingramcontent.com/pod-product-compliance
Lightning Source LLC
Chambersburg PA
CBHW060705280326
41933CB00012B/2305